Nudism At Home

by Glen McGinnis

Embracing Nudism at Home

Embracing nudism at home opens the doors to a realm of unparalleled comfort and liberation within the sanctuary of your personal space. It is like stepping into a tranquil oasis where the constraints of clothing fade away, allowing you to exist in a state of pure authenticity and freedom. Imagine waking up each morning to the soft glow of sunlight cascading through your windows, the gentle caress of the air on your skin creating a symphony of sensations that nourish your soul.

Nudism at home transcends mere nudity; it is a profound practice of shedding layers, both physical and emotional, and embracing the raw beauty of your natural self. Within the intimate confines of your living space, you are free to revel in the exquisite simplicity of being bare, unencumbered by the expectations of society. Every moment becomes a celebration of your true essence, a gentle reminder that beneath the facade of clothing lies a body that is inherently perfect and worthy of acceptance.

As you navigate your home in the nude, you become attuned to the subtle delights of existence – the coolness of the floor beneath your feet, the warmth of sunlight on your skin, the unrestricted movement that allows you to connect with your body in a way that feels profoundly authentic. This practice cultivates a profound sense of self-appreciation, nurturing a deep connection with your physical form and fostering a newfound appreciation for its innate beauty and uniqueness.

Whether you choose to explore nudism at home in solitude or with others who share your reverence for naturalness, the experience is one that can be profoundly empowering. It is a gentle invitation to strip away the layers of judgment and shame that society often imposes, and instead, embrace the purity and simplicity of your true self. Within the walls of your home, you are free to be wholly and unapologetically yourself – a beautiful, natural being deserving of love and acceptance exactly as you are.

So, immerse yourself in the serene tranquility of nudism at home. Embrace the freedom, comfort, and authenticity that come with shedding societal expectations and rediscovering the profound beauty of your unadorned self. In this sacred space, let go of inhibitions, bask in the peacefulness of simply being, and revel in the exquisite joy of existing in harmony with your true nature.

Understanding Body Positivity

In the realm of body positivity, there exists a serene oasis of self-acceptance and reverence for one's own physical form. It's like floating effortlessly in a tranquil pool of self-love, feeling the gentle ripples of unconditional acceptance caress your soul. Embracing body positivity is akin to embarking on a sacred journey of self-discovery, where every curve, scar, and imperfection is embraced with tender admiration.

As you delve deeper into the essence of body positivity, you will find yourself on a path of awakening, where you learn to honor and celebrate the beauty that resides within you. It's about recognizing that your body is not just a vessel, but a sacred temple that houses the essence of your being, deserving of nothing less than absolute reverence and gratitude.

In this serene sanctuary of self-compassion, the barometer of beauty is not dictated by societal norms or external standards, but by the pure essence of love and acceptance that emanates from within. It's about releasing yourself from the confines of comparison and judgment, and allowing yourself to bask in the glow of your own radiance, appreciating the unique tapestry of your body in all its raw, unfiltered beauty.

Embracing body positivity goes beyond the physical realm; it extends to nourishing your mental and emotional well-being, fostering a deep sense of self-worth and empowerment. It's an intimate dance of self-exploration and self-celebration, where you learn to honor your strengths and vulnerabilities alike, weaving them into a tapestry of self-love that is as intricate and beautiful as the night sky.

As you embark on this journey of self-discovery and self-acceptance, you will witness a transformation within yourself, a blossoming of confidence and self-assurance that radiates from the depths of your being. You will begin to see beauty not as a fixed image to attain, but as a fluid, ever-evolving expression of individuality that is inherently yours to embrace and celebrate.

So, immerse yourself in the gentle waters of body positivity, let the waves of self-acceptance and self-love wash over you, and remember that true beauty lies not in conformity, but in the raw, untamed essence of your authentic self. Embrace your body as

---

Understanding Body Positivity

In the realm of body positivity, there exists a serene oasis of self-acceptance and reverence for one's own physical form. It's like floating effortlessly in a tranquil pool of self-love, feeling the gentle ripples of unconditional acceptance caress your soul. Embracing body positivity is akin to embarking on a sacred journey of self-discovery, where every curve, scar, and imperfection is embraced with tender admiration.

As you delve deeper into the essence of body positivity, you will find yourself on a path of awakening, where you learn to honor and celebrate the beauty that resides within you. It's about recognizing that your body is not just a vessel, but a sacred temple that houses the essence of your being, deserving of nothing less than absolute reverence and gratitude.

In this serene sanctuary of self-compassion, the barometer of beauty is not dictated by societal norms or external standards, but by the pure essence of love and acceptance that emanates from within. It's about releasing yourself from the confines of comparison and judgment, and allowing yourself to bask in the glow of your own radiance, appreciating the unique tapestry of your body in all its raw, unfiltered beauty.

Embracing body positivity goes beyond the physical realm; it extends to nourishing your mental and emotional well-being, fostering a deep sense of self-worth and empowerment. It's an intimate dance of self-exploration and self-celebration, where you learn to honor your strengths and vulnerabilities alike, weaving them into a tapestry of self-love that is as intricate and beautiful as the night sky.

As you embark on this journey of self-discovery and self-acceptance, you will witness a transformation within yourself, a blossoming of confidence and self-assurance that radiates from the depths of your being. You will begin to see beauty not as a fixed image to attain, but as a fluid, ever-evolving expression of individuality that is inherently yours to embrace and celebrate.

So, immerse yourself in the gentle waters of body positivity, let the waves of self-acceptance and self-love wash over you, and remember that true beauty lies not in conformity, but in the raw, untamed essence of your authentic self. Embrace your body as the sacred vessel that carries your spirit through this journey called life, and adorn it with the colors of love, acceptance, and grace.

Creating a Comfortable Nudist Environment

In creating a comfortable nudist environment, the key is to focus on relaxation and acceptance. When it comes to embracing nudism at home, it's important to create a space where you feel at ease and free from judgment. Start by choosing areas in your home where you feel most comfortable being nude, whether it's the living room, bedroom, or even your backyard.

Consider factors like lighting, temperature, and furniture arrangement to enhance your comfort level. Soft lighting and warm colors can help set a relaxed mood, creating a cozy atmosphere that encourages you to let go of any inhibitions. Embrace the natural light streaming in through windows, casting a gentle glow that envelops you in a sense of tranquility.

When it comes to temperature, adjust it to your preference – whether you enjoy a warm and soothing environment or a cooler, refreshing atmosphere. Surround yourself with textiles that feel soft against your skin, such as plush rugs and silky blankets, enhancing the tactile experience of being nude in your space.

Create designated lounging areas that invite you to unwind and relax fully. Comfortable seating like oversized cushions or a plush couch beckon you to sink into a state of blissful serenity. Arrange your furniture in a way that promotes an open and airy feel, allowing you to move freely and embrace the liberating sensation of being unencumbered by clothing.

Engage in activities that bring you joy and enhance your sense of well-being while in your nudist space. Whether it's listening to soothing music, practicing gentle yoga poses, or immersing yourself in a good book, let yourself fully unwind and embrace the present moment. The key is to prioritize your comfort and self-care, allowing yourself to revel in the beauty of your natural state.

By cultivating a welcoming and accepting environment in your home, you can fully embrace the nudist lifestyle and experience a profound sense of freedom and self-acceptance. Embrace the beauty of your body and the serenity of being nude, allowing yourself to bask in the simplicity and purity of the moment. In this relaxed setting, you will find a deep connection to yourself and a renewed sense of peace and contentment.

Nudism and Family Dynamics

Family dynamics are a complex tapestry, woven with threads of love, understanding, and shared experiences. When it comes to nudism and family, navigating this delicate balance requires open communication and a willingness to embrace new perspectives.

Introducing the concept of nudism to your family can be akin to delicately planting a seed of understanding and acceptance. It's crucial to approach the topic with sensitivity and empathy, allowing each family member to express their thoughts and concerns openly. By creating a safe space for dialogue, you pave the way for a deeper connection rooted in trust and respect.

Nudism, at its core, promotes body positivity and self-acceptance. By baring it all together, families can cultivate a sense of unity and appreciation for the diverse beauty of the human form. This shared experience reinforces bonds and fosters a culture of acceptance within the family unit.

In a world inundated with societal norms and expectations, nudism offers a refreshing perspective on the concept of nudity. By embracing nudity as a family, you challenge conventional beliefs and cultivate a healthy attitude towards the body. Children raised in a nudist environment are more likely to develop a positive body image and a profound sense of self-confidence.

Participating in nudist activities as a family can create a treasure trove of memories etched in laughter, freedom, and connection. This shared experience not only strengthens emotional ties but also enriches the family's collective identity.

In the tapestry of family life, nudism adds a vibrant thread of liberation and authenticity. By shedding inhibitions and embracing vulnerability, families can forge a deep sense of intimacy and trust. Through nudism, families can rewrite the narrative around nudity and instill a sense of reverence for the natural beauty of the human body.

In conclusion, integrating nudism into family life is a journey of self-discovery, empathy, and growth. By embarking on this path together, families cultivate a culture of acceptance, understanding, and unwavering love. In the shared embrace of nudity, families find not only freedom but also a profound connection that transcends words.

Open Communication in Nudist Families

In nudist families, open communication is the cornerstone that builds strong relationships and a sense of understanding and acceptance among family members. It's a way of fostering a supportive and nurturing environment where everyone feels comfortable expressing themselves without inhibition or fear of judgment.

When discussing nudism with children, parents should approach the conversation with honesty and openness, creating a space where questions can be asked freely and answers given without reservation. Encouraging open dialogue helps children to develop a healthy attitude towards nudity and to see it as a natural and normal part of life.

Mutual respect for each other's boundaries and preferences is essential within nudist families. By openly discussing and acknowledging each family member's comfort levels, everyone can feel heard and understood, fostering a sense of trust and acceptance within the family unit.

Nudism can be a beautiful way for families to bond and connect on a deeper level, but it's important to navigate any challenges that may arise with patience and understanding. By building a strong foundation of communication and trust, nudist families can create a harmonious and supportive environment where everyone feels valued and accepted for who they are.

Nudism and Privacy

Nudism, a lifestyle that thrives on the freedom of being in the raw, places a high value on privacy within its community. The concept of privacy among nudists is not merely a matter of physical boundaries but a deep-rooted culture of respect and consent that permeates every interaction.

In the world of nudism, privacy is sacred, just as the gentle rustle of leaves in a secluded forest glade. Nudists cherish personal space and uphold it with the utmost care, recognizing the importance of creating a safe and comfortable environment for all. This commitment to privacy is underpinned by a profound belief in the power of enthusiastic consent and clear communication.

Within nudist circles, the mantra of "ask first, respect always" guides every interaction. Whether it's seeking permission before capturing a moment in a photograph or initiating any form of physical contact, nudists navigate their interactions with the sensitivity of a butterfly alighting on a flower petal. This emphasis on mutual respect fosters a sense of trust and camaraderie, where individuals can shed their inhibitions along with their clothing, secure in the knowledge that their boundaries will be honored.

Designated nudist spaces, such as serene beaches and welcoming resorts, serve as sanctuaries where privacy and freedom intertwine like the branches of a sun-dappled grove. In these havens, nudists find solace in the knowledge that they can bask in the warmth of acceptance without fear of judgment or intrusion. These spaces are sacred ground, where the whisper of the wind carries the essence of liberation and the embrace of privacy envelopes each individual like a comforting shawl.

The art of navigating privacy in nudism is a delicate dance, where the graceful interplay of personal comfort and mutual respect takes center stage. It is a lifestyle that celebrates the beauty of individuality while also cherishing the harmony that arises from honoring the privacy and well-being of all community members. In the world of nudism, privacy is not merely a concept but a way of being—a gentle reminder that in the dance of life, every soul deserves the space to move freely and authentically, unencumbered by the weight of judgment or intrusion.

Challenging Social Stigmas

In a world where societal norms often dictate how we should live and present ourselves, nudists find themselves facing unique challenges and misconceptions. The practice of nudism, often misunderstood and stigmatized, is actually rooted in a deep sense of body acceptance, freedom, and connection to nature.

It can be daunting to challenge these deeply ingrained social stigmas, but nudists are determined to live authentically and embrace their bodies with confidence and pride. By rejecting societal expectations and choosing to live nudist lifestyles, individuals are making a powerful statement about self-acceptance and individuality.

Education and open-mindedness play crucial roles in breaking down these stigmas. By engaging in respectful conversations and sharing personal experiences, nudists can help others understand the true essence of nudism: it's not about seeking attention or being scandalous, but rather about feeling liberated and comfortable in one's own skin.

Nudism offers numerous benefits, including promoting body positivity, improving self-esteem, and fostering a stronger connection to the natural world. By embodying these values and living their truth, nudists can inspire others to challenge their own biases and prejudices, ultimately leading to a more inclusive and understanding society.

So, let's continue to walk confidently along the path of nudism, knowing that each step we take towards self-acceptance and liberation is a step towards a more open-minded and compassionate world for all. Embrace your body, embrace your truth, and let's continue to challenge those societal stigmas, one conversation at a time.

Nudism is not merely about shedding clothes; it's about shedding inhibitions and embracing a sense of freedom that is often lacking in our society. By allowing ourselves to be vulnerable in our natural state, we can truly connect with ourselves and the world around us on a deeper level.

The misconceptions surrounding nudism stem from a lack of understanding and exposure. Through education and open dialogue, we can work towards dispelling these myths and encouraging a more accepting and inclusive attitude towards nudist practices.

As we navigate the complexities of societal expectations and norms, nudists stand as a symbol of defiance against conformity and a beacon of self-acceptance. By choosing to live authentically and unapologetically, they challenge others to question their own beliefs and biases.

In a world that often judges and criticizes based on external appearances, nudists remind us that true beauty and confidence come from within. Embracing our natural selves without shame or hesitation, we can learn to love and appreciate our bodies for the unique vessels they are.

So let's continue to embrace the nudist lifestyle with courage and resilience, knowing that by doing so, we are not only honoring ourselves but also paving the way for a more tolerant and understanding world for generations to come.

Nudism and Healthy Living

Incorporating nudism into your lifestyle can truly be a liberating experience, allowing you to connect with yourself and the world around you in a more genuine and unencumbered way.

When you strip away the layers of clothing and embrace your natural state, you are giving yourself permission to let go of societal expectations and pressures related to body image. Without the confines of clothing, you can truly come to appreciate and accept your body for what it is, unique and beautiful in its own way.

Nudism promotes a sense of body positivity and self-acceptance that can have a profound impact on your overall well-being. By basking in the freedom of being naked, you can cultivate a deeper sense of self-confidence and inner peace, knowing that you are enough just as you are.

Moreover, going au naturel allows your skin to breathe and thrive, potentially decreasing the likelihood of skin irritations and promoting better overall hygiene. Embracing nudity can lead to healthier skin, improved circulation, and a greener approach to personal care.

Participating in nudist activities often involves spending time outdoors, connecting with natural elements, and soaking up the sun's rays. This exposure to nature can help reduce stress, elevate your mood, and create a sense of harmony between your body and the surrounding environment.

In essence, nudism is not just about shedding your clothes; it's about shedding the layers of societal conditioning and allowing yourself to exist authentically and unapologetically. Embracing nudism can be a journey towards greater self-acceptance, body positivity, and a more profound connection to yourself and the world around you. Go ahead, bask in the freedom of your natural state and let your worries fade away as you embrace the peaceful serenity of nudism. Feel the sun's warm rays on your skin, listen to the soothing sounds of nature, and revel in the beauty of being truly and unapologetically yourself.

Nudism and Self-Acceptance

In a world that often tells us to hide our bodies and conform to unrealistic standards, nudism can be a powerful practice in self-acceptance. Embracing nudism allows individuals to connect with their bodies in a way that promotes self-love and confidence.

When we shed our clothes and embrace our natural state, we are accepting ourselves exactly as we are, without any need for shame or judgment. Nudism encourages us to appreciate our bodies for all their uniqueness and beauty, regardless of societal expectations.

Through nudism, we learn to celebrate our bodies as they are, without resorting to comparisons or self-criticism. We recognize that every body is different and that diversity is something to be honored and embraced.

By practicing nudism, we can cultivate a deeper sense of self-acceptance and self-love. We begin to see ourselves not through the lens of societal norms or beauty standards, but through a lens of authenticity and appreciation for our own bodies.

Nudism teaches us that our bodies are not something to be hidden or ashamed of, but something to be cherished and honored. It allows us to let go of insecurities and embrace our bodies with confidence and grace.

Ultimately, nudism can be a powerful tool in fostering self-acceptance and body positivity. It encourages us to love ourselves exactly as we are, unapologetically and authentically. Through nudism, we can learn to embrace and celebrate our bodies in all their natural glory.

By recognizing the beauty and uniqueness of each individual body, nudism helps us to celebrate our differences and promote a culture of body acceptance. It allows us to break free from the constraints of societal beauty standards and embrace our bodies with a sense of freedom and confidence.

Nudism also promotes a deeper connection to nature and the world around us. By experiencing the natural elements on our skin without barriers, we can feel more in tune with the earth and our place within it. This connection can bring a sense of peace and grounding that is hard to find in a world that often feels disconnected from the natural world.

As we continue to practice nudism, we may find that our self-esteem and body image improve as we learn to love and accept ourselves just as we are. We begin to see our bodies not as objects of scrutiny, but as vessels of strength, beauty, and resilience. This shift in perspective can lead to a more positive relationship with ourselves and a greater sense of self-worth.

In embracing nudism, we embrace ourselves fully and authentically, letting go of the need to conform to external standards and instead focusing on our own inner sense of beauty and worth. It is a practice that challenges us to be vulnerable, to be brave, and to love ourselves unconditionally.

Nudism as a Lifestyle Choice

As nudism continues to gain popularity and acceptance, more and more individuals are finding solace in the freedom of shedding their clothing and embracing their natural state of being. It's not just about baring our skin; it goes much deeper, touching the core of our authenticity and self-acceptance.

Choosing a nudist lifestyle is a profound personal journey that allows us to break free from societal constraints and embrace a more natural, unfiltered way of living. With each layer of clothing shed, there's a shedding of inhibitions, judgments, and insecurities, leading to a deeper connection with ourselves and the world around us.

Nudism isn't just about being nude; it's a philosophy of openness, acceptance, and liberation. It's about feeling the sun and wind directly on our skin, connecting with nature in its purest form, and experiencing a sense of freedom that comes from embracing our bodies without reservation. Many nudists describe a feeling of lightness and joy when practicing nudism, as if a weight has been lifted off their shoulders.

Living a nudist lifestyle also fosters a unique sense of community and belonging. Nudist communities provide a safe space where everyone is accepted and celebrated for who they are, regardless of their shape or size. In this non-judgmental environment, there's a shared understanding and acceptance of the human body in all its forms, fostering a deep sense of unity and camaraderie among its members.

Ultimately, nudism as a lifestyle choice is a path to greater self-expression, self-acceptance, and connection – both to ourselves and to others. It's a way of living that celebrates the beauty of the human body in its natural state, promoting body positivity, authenticity, and a profound sense of freedom. If you're considering nudism as a lifestyle choice, remember that it's not just about taking off your clothes – it's about embracing a way of living that honors your true self and the beauty of being exactly who you are.

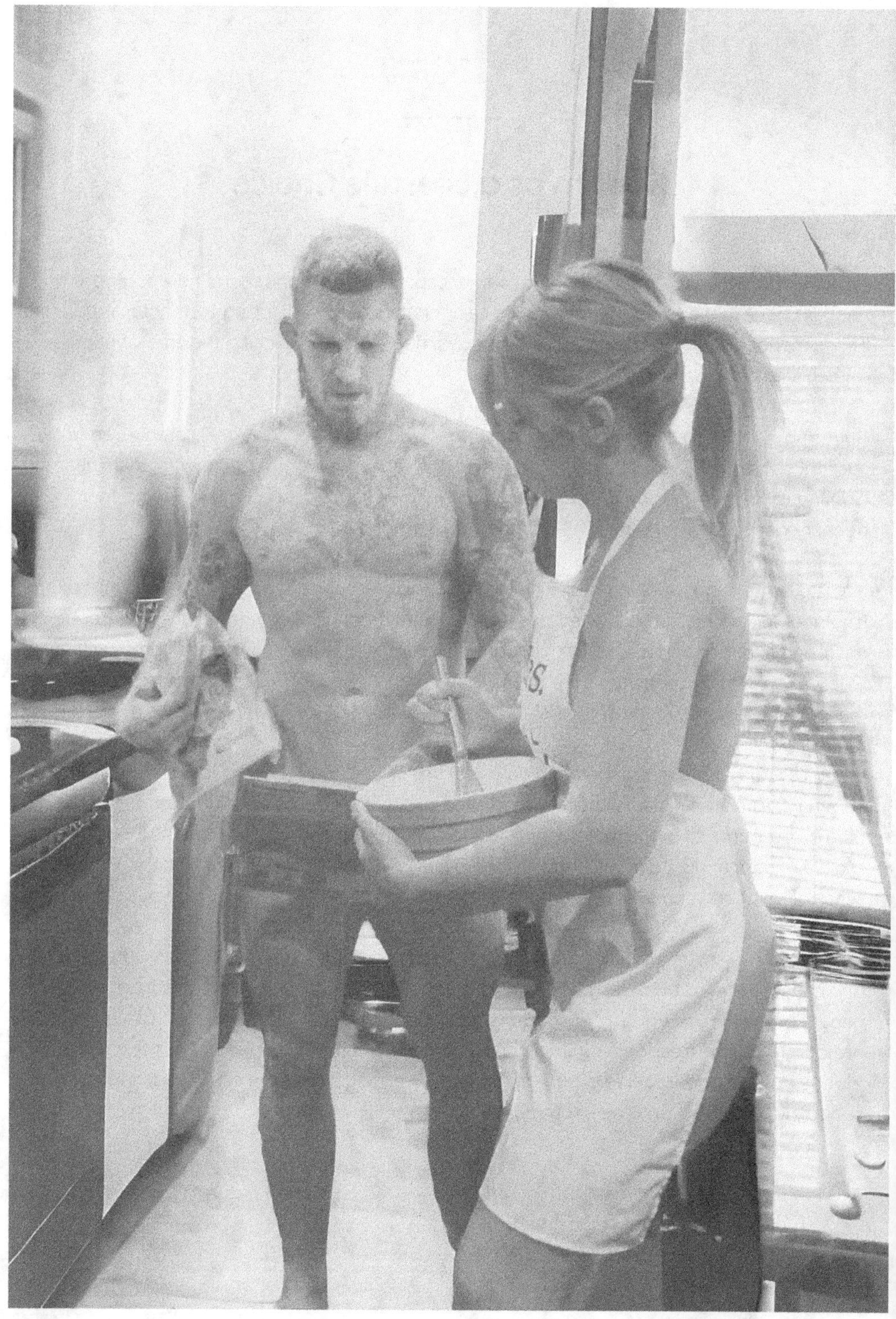